Holistic Insights

For

Everyday Wellness

Volume 1

Dedicated to every living soul who has helped us to become who we are today.

Table of Contents

Foreword

First of all thank yourself for diving into this health inspired literature. You deserve to thrive and enjoy every day to the fullest. Knowledge is shared and the cycle continues. I hope this book inspires you to continue learning about yourself and your full potential.

Ways to Improve the Mind Body Connection

What is Mind Body Medicine?

Mind body medicine can be defined as the capacity to have a positive influence on mental function, emotions, and physiology. Mind body medicine encompasses a wide range of therapies such as meditation, guided imagery, hatha yoga, Qigong, and Tai Chi.

There is solid scientific evidence regarding the benefits of mind-body approaches over the last 40 years.[1] Mind body medicine recognizes the need for us to exercise and act as one unit, which in turn can add many benefits to our health and how we live life.

The first studies were conducted at Yale and Rockefeller Universities in animals. Yogis of India were also studied and found to have significant control over autonomic nervous system functions such as heart rate and pain perception.[2]

Your hormones and your immune system can also be affected in a positive way by practicing some type of mind body exercise. Psychoneuroimmunology (the connection of the mind and the immune system via the nervous system) and psychoneuroendocrinology (the connection between the mind and your hormones via the nervous system) have been shown to be affected by exercise. The same neurotransmitters that send messages to the central nervous system also send to the endocrine system.[3]

A Review of Anatomy and Physiology

Autonomic Nervous System – Our fight or flight system, controls our cardiac muscle, smooth muscle, and glandular epithelial cells (sweat glands, pancreas, liver). This is the system that tells us whether to fight the bear or run in fear.

Limbic System – Located in the cerebral cortex, deals with emotional memory. Good and bad memories ares stored here and can trigger reactions throughout the body.

Hypothalamus and Pineal Gland — Located in the brain, has influence on hormones and sleeping patterns (pineal gland), and is considered to be a key link between the mind and the body.

Yoga for Strengthening the Mind/Body Connection

Yoga is an exercise that is thousands of years old and began in India. It involves holding physical postures, breathing techniques, meditation, and relaxation of yourself. Prior to the first time I tried hatha yoga, my thoughts were along the lines of, "This isn't going to be that hard," "I've stretched plenty of times prior," and "#1 student!" But alas, I was wrong, and it was a hard, fun, self-satisfying, peaceful workout which really gave me a chance to work on my balance and centering my mind.

The practice of yoga has been shown to significantly decrease finger pain during activity and improved finger range of motion in osteoarthritis patients.[4] It is also used to promote self-awareness, emotional stability, and peace of mind. In addition, yoga has been shown to improve communication, attention, energy, and focus, as well as enhance feelings of overall wellness and well-being.[5]

Biofeedback at a Glance

I want to touch briefly on this subject, but mainly biofeedback involves using instruments and devices to monitor bodily activity and induce a state of calmness. It has been used in management of diseases such as hypertension, stroke, and Systemic Lupus Erythematosus, or SLE.

TaiJiQuan for Mind and Body Enhancement

TaiJiQuan or Tai Chi Chuan was developed around the 1300s, but Qigong breathing exercises have been around for a few thousand years. They are slow moving, meditative exercises that focus on breathing and attention. Qigong is more focused on circulation and vitality, while Tai Chi is focused more on meditative movement and self defense. They are both used to inspire inner awareness and increase longevity, as both are needed in order to progress to higher levels.

Benefits of Tai Chi include:

- Increased relaxation
- Increased focus
- Decreased blood pressure
- Improved lymphatic function

- Improved immune system
- Promotion of alpha/beta wave activity

Meditation

Meditation is a method to focus on your breathing and inner awareness. There are multiple methods of meditation but abdominal or solar plexus breathing is the main concept amongst all.

Work up to meditating for longer periods. It's not meant to be conquered in a day. According to the National Center For Complementary and Alternative Medicine (NCCAM), meditation has been used for:

- Anxiety
- Pain
- Depression
- Stress
- Insomnia
- Physical or emotional symptoms that may be associated with chronic illnesses (such as heart disease, HIV/AIDS, and cancer) and their treatment.

This is a small list and anyone who wants to rest their mind and focus on their breathing will benefit from meditation.

Integrate Mind Body Training into Your Routine

This is a brief introduction into the reasons why mind body medicine is important. Make sure to train under a knowledgeable teacher so that you learn proper technique. Know that mind body medicine entails a variety of different exercises and techniques, and really it comes down to whichever methods work best for you, as long as you take that first step forward!

References and Sources:

1,2,3,Rakel, D. Faass, N. 2006. *Complementary Medicine in Clinical Practice.* Jones and Barlett Publishers, Inc.
Thibodeau, G. *Anatomy and Physiology*, Mosby Inc.
4,5,6, Complementary and alternative exercises for management of osteoarthritis. *Arthritis.* 2011;2011:364319. Epub 2011 Jul 25.

Body Mind Health: The Hypothalamus

Hippopotamus? Ah, hypothalamus!

You know, there are a lot of interesting parts and regions in the brain that we'll be studying for years to come, and the hypothalamus can be tossed into that group (don't toss it too hard!). The hypothalamus plays a huge role in the following areas[1]:

- Hunger

- Mood and feelings

- Sexual drive

- Sleep

- Temperature

- Thirst

- The releasing of hormones

It is located just around the center of the brain and is surrounded by various glands. The hypothalamus weighs around seven grams, and is located beneath the thalamus, which is responsible for functions such as pain, temperature, and crude touch. The hypothalamus has been considered a major link between the mind and the body, providing a route for emotions to express themselves through the body.

Functions of the Hypothalamus

The hypothalamus plays a major role in secreting releasing hormones, which are responsible for, as you may have guessed, releasing hormones. It doesn't do it directly, but rather signals different glands, primarily the pituitary gland, which then releases the hormone when it is needed. You can view it as the general

who gives the order to fire the cannon ball. Some of the hormones released by the hypothalamus include:

- Corticotropin-releasing hormone–affects adrenal glands and cortisol

- Growth hormone-releasing hormone and Growth hormone-inhibiting hormone

- Prolactin releasing hormone–plays a role in breast milk secretion and menstruation

The hypothalamus also plays a role keeping you awake during the day, as clinical data suggests it plays a role in sleepiness disorders.[2] Its neurons (nerve cells) connect with the autonomic centers for the functions of sweating and shivering. In Traditional Chinese Medicine, we attribute the control of pores and temperature to what we call "wei qi," or your outside defense qi (pronounced "chee"). This type of qi also plays a role in immunity, protecting you from outside infectious agents.

Mind Body Health and the Hypothalamus

In stressful situations, the hypothalamus serves an important function. Emotional memory from the limbic system (which stores good and bad feelings of past memories) can communicate and send nerve impulses to the hypothalamus. This leads to increased stimulation of the pituitary gland and an increase in hormones secreted into the body. This is an interesting link between nerve impulses and hormones, because it tells us that our feelings and thoughts can really affect how our body operates. The hypothalamus can take over your pituitary gland and affect every cell in your body if put into a situation where your survival is in danger![3]

Acupuncture has been shown to promote positive interaction in the hypothalamus, being able to increase or decrease signal stimulation.[4] It is interesting that acupuncture can affect the hypothalamus in such a way as to balance it, because acupuncture naturally helps to bring the body to a state of relaxation and homeostasis (stability).

Meditation has also been shown to have a positive impact on factors such as cortisol secretion and the hypothalamic-pituitary-adrenocortical system, which is the connection between the hypothalamus, the pituitary gland, and your adrenal system, and which is responsible for adrenaline[5].

The hypothalamus is a fascinating area of the brain that plays a vital role in our lives. Holistic medicine encompasses healing all bodily and mental systems in order to achieve optimal wellness. Please feel free to read the first part of the Body Mind Health series on the pineal gland, and stay tuned for more posts on the journey into the mind and body.

References

1. Medline Plus Medicine. 2011. Hypothalamus. Retrieved March 30, 2012 from *Medline Plus*. Retrieved March 30, 2012 from
http://www.nlm.nih.gov/medlineplus/ency/article/002380.htm

2, 3. Thibodeau, G. *Anatomy and Physiology*, Mosby Inc, 2003

4,5. Brand S, Holsboer-Trachsler E, Naranjo JR, Schmidt S. Influence of Mindfulness Practice on Cortisol and Sleep in Long-Term and Short-Term Meditators. *Neuropsychobiology*. 2012 Feb 24;65(3):109-118

Body Mind Health: The Pineal Gland

Your Third Eye

Why is it called the third eye? Because of its connection to regulating so many bodily functions and utilizing the natural sun to regulate the body. It works with the hypothalamus to help regulate certain body functions that we don't think about, such as when we are hungry. Your third eye is much more than just one gland, but a series of systems keeping us connected to the universe. It has been associated with intuition, spirituality, and a higher level of consciousness in different cultures and schools of thought throughout time. Sometimes it is easy to forget, in this fast paced society with refrigerators, heaters, and air conditioners, that we are connected to this earth and universe. When we begin acknowledging this and make changes to live a lifestyle more balanced with nature, we will reap the many health benefits gained and live a more fulfilled life.

Melatonin as an Antioxidant

Your pineal gland secretes a hormone called melatonin that helps you to go to sleep. Melatonin is also a free radical scavenger, with the ability to fight free radicals. This is really amazing because melatonin acts as an antioxidant to protect your body, and it's ability to detoxify the hydroxyl radical (-OH) and has been shown to be higher than vitamin C or vitamin E.[1] This is why I tell people that you have power to heal within yourself because you have healing cells!

Seasonal affective disorder (SAD) is a condition associated with severe depression during the winter when the days are shorter. Thus, current research suggests that melatonin plays a role in this disorder. Traditional Chinese Medicine has always considered weather and seasons to play a significant role in disease and wellness. Even a cloudy day can affect your physical and mental behaviors!

Current scientific data indicates that visual cues received by the pineal gland help to determine the day length, as well as the different phases of the moon (lunar cycle). The pineal gland assists your biological clocks. Your biological clocks are cells that interact on the molecular level, all synchronized by a master clock. This master clock is located in an area call the suprachiasmatic nucleus,[2] which is where the left and right optic nerves cross.

TCM and Natural Cycles

In Traditional Chinese Medicine (TCM), there are a number of different systems in place that help regulate your body with nature. For instance, in what is known as the horary cycle, each organ has a certain time of the day where its energy is flowing more potently than at other times.

It is also natural that the daytime represents yang and nighttime represents yin, and they both work in balance to preside over their respective time periods. There are certain types of qi responsible for the opening and shutting of the eyes, helping the mind to remain at rest, regulating menstruation, and helping the body to perform other natural functions that we don't usually think about.

Sources and References

1. Tamura H, Takasaki A, Taketani T, Tanabe M, Kizuka F, Lee L, Tamura I, Maekawa R, Aasada H, Yamagata Y, Sugino N.The role of melatonin as an antioxidant in the follicle. *J Ovarian Res*. 2012 Jan 26;5:5.

2. National Institute of General Medical Sciences. 2012. *Circadian Rhythms Fact Sheet*. Retrieved March 27th, 2012 from

http://www.nigms.nih.gov/Education/Factsheet_CircadianRhythms.htm

5 Ways to Live More Natural, Organic, and Healthy

While hanging out watching Tim Tebow do his "magic" on the field, I came up with the idea of writing a few tips on how I've taken a more holistic approach to living, and it may be beneficial to you as well. It is my belief that everything in life is a journey, and if you are not great at something, don't worry, you can always improve. Anyone who tells you otherwise is what we sometimes call a "hater," which is someone who flagrantly demeans your effort or offers negative criticism for no reason. But don't worry, the main goal is to try to find out what works best for you and do things one step at a time.

1. *Try using lemon as deodorant*

Even though more evidence is needed to support the theory that antiperspirant deodorants may cause diseases such as breast cancer, it doesn't hurt to use something natural from your own backyard or local farmer. You may not want to use it if you have open wounds or cuts under your arms because it may sting. But why use a product from an industry that remains largely unregulated, such as the cosmetic industry? If you can use a lemon to achieve great smelling results, why not?

2. *Go to bed earlier*

In Traditional Chinese Medicine theory, it is recommended that you go to bed at a decent time, preferably before 11pm. My teacher used to say if you miss the boat, then you miss the boat. I became so amazed with Chinese Medicine because of their foresight into human physiology. The body is regulated by certain glands, one of these being the pineal gland. It is located in the diencephalon of the brain, above the brain stem, and is responsible for regulating natural functions such as inducing sleep by producing melatonin and waking us up. It is also known as our "third eye" and is being studied as a major connection in the mind-body relationship.

It is important to keep to our natural rhythm because it is wired into your body to follow the rhythm of nature. A 2001 study in the *Journal of the National Cancer Institute* found an increased risk of breast cancer associated with night shift work and light exposure at night.[3] I always say go to sleep early and wake up early to enjoy the day!

3. Sneak organic foods into your diet if you're not doing so already

If you have the ability and the means to fill your entire fridge with organic food, then go for it. However, if money is an issue, as it is for most people, then there are some ways to at least incorporate more organic foods into your shopping cart. First, check out your local farmer's market; you will find many deals on great veggies and fruits. Get to know the growers and their products, and learn recipes to make soups, which are healthy and very cost efficient. Trader Joe's and Whole Foods offer many brands comparable to their non-organic counterparts for just a little bit more money, sometimes just by a couple of cents. Items that are typically very reasonably priced include organic peanut/almond butter, jelly and jams, organic whole wheat spaghetti, brown rice, apples, carrots, greens, and frozen veggies. They have a good selection of fruits and veggies, but prices can vary on these items and run a bit on the high side.

4. Take a walk and move

I'm a fan of walking, especially since it's a lot easier on the knees. However, you don't have to just walk in the mornings or when you get home from work. You can do both, and you can also take a walk during your lunch and during your breaks. The duration of your walk is up to you, but I think splitting your walks into 10 minutes each is definitely doable. If you did that three to four times a day, you would gain 30-40 minutes of exercise from just those small activities.

5. Put down the sodas, pick up the water

Drinking enough water was one of the first things I really enjoyed changing in my life. I decided to do this back in my undergrad days at Cal Poly Pomona to save a couple dollars on groceries and stay healthy. Ever since, I've always kept myself well hydrated and it feels great.

I'm always improving and looking for new ways to keep to my living style in this ever changing world, and as things become more hectic and fast-paced, it becomes more important to find out what works for us and put it into action. What have you done to make the direction of your life more healthy and natural?

References
1. Namer M, Luporsi E, Gligorov J, Lokiec F, Spielmann M. The use of deodorants/antiperspirants does not constitute a risk factor for breast cancer. Bull Cancer. 2008 Sep;95(9):871-80. Retrieved from http://www.jle.com/en/revues/medecine/bdc/e-docs/00/04/40/D1/resume.phtml
2. Mirick DK, Davis S, Thomas DB. Antiperspirant use and the risk of breast cancer.J Natl Cancer Inst. 2002 Oct 16;94(20):1578-80.
3. Davis S, Mirick DK, Stevens RG. Night shift work, light at night, and risk of breast cancer. J Natl Cancer Inst. 2001 Oct 17;93(20):1557-62.

A Smoothie Recipe to Lose Weight and Build Endurance

I don't think anyone could turn down a good shake or smoothie. For this idea, I actually have to thank my sister. She is also conscious of living a healthy, holistic lifestyle and is a good model for people to learn from. You'll receive few stares when you tell them that this is a spinach, peanut butter, and banana shake. At first you may think, "A spinach shake?" That was my first impression too, since I was so accustomed to having my spinach a certain way. Nevertheless, it was one of the best shakes that I've tried and now I'm passing it along to you, thanks to my sis and whoever passed it along to her! So here is what you need:

- ○ 1-1/2 to 2 bananas, organic recommended but make do with what you have.

- ○ 2 cups of spinach (raw or cooked) – Originally the recipe called for uncooked spinach but I used cooked spinach to help remove goitrogens. There is research into the effects of goitrogens on thyroid function and hypothyroidism and I'm still gathering some more information supporting their negative effects. However, just for safe measure, I boil my spinach. On top of that, in Chinese Medicine we believe that foods should generally be warm when consumed. This adds a bit of warmth to the shake and it still tastes great. You should boil the spinach for about five minutes. If you would like to add more spinach, be my guest.

- ○ 1/2 cup of alfalfa sprouts – Adding more greens to the mix, this is a great way to add nutrition without sacrificing taste. Since alfalfa sprouts do carry quite a bit of water, try not to overdo it or you may have a water-logged shake.

- ○ 2 tablespoons of almond/sunflower/peanut butter – Add a little protein to the mix. Not only does it give you a nice eight grams of it, but it makes the drink taste great as well.

It is recommended that you use almond or sunflower spread optimally, but hey, if you can only afford peanut butter then run with it, I ain't hatin' (which means not frowning upon)! The more organic/natural you can get it, the better. If you can make your own, that would be optimal.

o   A dash of Cinnamon – Cinnamon in Traditional Chinese Medicine is considered a great herb! It used in Chinese herbal formulations for colds with sweating, post stroke recovery, and muscle pain. I dash a bit into the spinach while it's boiling so that they both get about five minutes of boiling time. Also, cinnamon is granulated so you can boil it in some type of cloth and let the cinnamon compounds soak into the spinach

o   8-12 ounces of water: Yup, you guessed it. Aqua. The real deal. You don't want to put in too much water because then it becomes more liquid than smooth, but you also don't want to add too little because it won't blend, my friend. So find the right mix for you; I usually use around one half to three quarters of a 16 ounce water bottle.

Mix all of the ingredients blending the cooked spinach with the water first to help break everything up. Drink, enjoy, and use it as a pre- or post-workout drink. This is only a general guideline, so feel free to try new variations to switch it up.

My only concern about this is that I try to eat foods that are local grown. I also now understand why people started the barter system (will work or trade you for bananas). Do you have any ideas on how to replace the bananas so that this smoothie still tastes great? Do you have any ideas for a good smoothie yourself?

To be or not to be...Happy

When you think of the word happy, what is the first thought that comes to mind? It probably might not be a thought; it could even be a reaction as simple as a smile when you're thinking about the word. I thought of the idea about writing this post from a video my father made. He is a musician in Germany, and his slogan was always, "Don't worry, be happy, and everything will work out." Sometimes when your life is crumbling around you it may be hard to keep positive, and really that is the most important thing you can do. According to Merriam-Webster.com, happiness is defined as "a state of well-being and contentment." The CDC estimates that one out of 10 US adults report depression,1 which doesn't include the unreported cases, as well as the depression levels found in teens and children.

According to the CDC, the individuals with a higher risk of depression include:

- Persons 45-64 years of age

- Women

- Blacks, Hispanics, non-Hispanic persons of other races or multiple races

- Persons with less than a high school education

- Those previously married

- Individuals unable to work or unemployed

- Persons without health insurance coverage

The last two bullet points I think stand out, especially since we are going through economic difficulties and healthcare is major topic amongst all Americans.

There are things that we can and can't change, and ultimately, sometimes the only thing you can change is how you view the situation.

What are some of the ways I keep myself happy?

- I take walks to the park, to the mountains, and to run my errands.

- I talk to family members or friends, or participate in online discussions and forums.

- I meditate and practice my deep breathing. I don't think about happy thoughts, I feel happy emotions. This includes doing my Tai Chi routine.

- I seek counseling or professional help. There is nothing to be ashamed about, and ask yourself who would a psychologist go to when they need help? Another psychologist.

- I write out what I'm feeling, which then turns to a game plan for the future and a motivational message to myself.

- I listen to motivational speakers, read motivational quotes and poems, and Google "motivation."

- I eat healthy, because crappy eating will make you feel like…well, crap.

- I exercise, which I know may sound repetitive but God made it for a reason, and so far it's one of my best tools.

What are some ways you try to keep yourself motivated and happy?

Remember to consult your primary healthcare provider if you feel that you may be suffering from symptoms of depression or other serious mental health issues.

References

1. Division of Adult and Community Health. 2011. CDC Data & Statistics. Retrieved January 10, 2011 from http://www.cdc.gov/features/dsdepression/

2. merriam-webster.com

5 Tips for Healthy Weight Loss

Losing weight can be a hard challenge. It can also be the most motivating and inspiring thing to happen in your life. When I began to really focus on my health and wanted to lose weight in college, I was determined. I was tired of the past ridicule, I was tired of not being able to date the type of women that I enjoyed company with, and I was tired of not being the person I knew that I could be. So I began my fitness journey while I was living at my fraternity house (we're not all beer guzzling Neanderthals, just a few of us), altering my diet and creating a workout plan. Six months later, I was 55 pounds lighter.

When you're overweight and don't feel good about yourself, the first thing you're most likely to say to yourself is, "Eh, I need to start losing some pounds." You are not alone. In fact, Americans spent over 120 billion dollars on weight loss products in 2009 and that number is only on the rise.[1] Diabetes has become a national health concern for millions of Americans, and there are many other diseases associated with being overweight.

So I decided to write this blog post to inspire you, to tell you that losing weight is not impossible; you just have to know and feel what you are doing is right. These are some tips that I have gained and still keep to this day.

1. Stick To The Basics

This is one of my favorites. I'm not a fan of fad diets at all. There will always be a new hype or "super supplement" to lose weight. What about the old way? Fruits and vegetables (go organic, if you're going, then do it right!); exercises such as tai chi, yoga, soccer, and swimming; good rest; correct portions of food, including cutting back on the Mickey-D's; and eating lots of soups and salads. Instead of focusing on new products on the market, start focusing on different ways to motivate yourself and your weight loss efforts will be doubled. I know sometimes we may get bored of doing the same exercises, eating the same food everyday, and going to the same gym, so switch it up and spice up your routine.

One last tip on new age remedies. Learning is an ongoing process, so new concepts that you learn that can be beneficial to your health can be positive. For instance, as acupuncturists we educate our patients on not consuming foods that are too cold and instead to eat warmer foods (temperature-wise) as well as foods that are easily digestible. In Chinese Medicine theory, we believe that to lose weight you want to move your qi and keep it circulating, and heat does that. If you consume something too cold, we believe it slows down the body's metabolism. Soups and salads go great together because they balance themselves out. Drinking room temperature water can a very positive benefit in your efforts. Is it necessary to purchase the newest weight loss gimmick to apply this to your life? No, just stick to the basics.

2. Get Help

You'll be surprised at who'll be willing to help you achieve your goals. Let your family and friends know so that they can support you, and who knows, you may even gain a workout buddy. But remember, you are doing this for yourself. There are many healthcare and wellness professionals here to help you achieve your goals.

3. Stay Positive

Stay positive! I say this for everything, for weight loss, diseases, or financial problems—stay positive. Life will work itself out if you just put in the work and have a goal set in mind. Yes, you will make mistakes. Yes, you may have a few days where you don't feel like you can put in 100%. Get back on that horse and keep riding. Even if you fall off, the sooner you get back on, the easier it will be to get back to your routine.

4. Use Goals and Measurements

There are many weight loss goal trackers and ways to measure your progress. The one I have used for over 10 years is from www.fitday.com and it is still around. You are able to track calorie intake, carbohydrates/fats/proteins (especially if you're diabetic it's good to monitor your carbohydrate intake), as well workouts and calories burned on average. Then you can look at the data weekly and monthly to track any trends you may have. This is very important because it's too hard to track your food intake by just using your memory. Having data on hand will give you a new perspective, and if you do it once, you'll have a better idea of how to eat just in case you can't track your food intake in the future. Just Google "fitness tracker" and try the one that works best for you.

5. Realize It Takes Time

It took some time to put on the weight, and now it is going to take time to take it off. Unfortunately, it may take more time to take of then it did to put it on, but that's life. Losing weight is a transformation process, and through that change it's important to reflect on yourself and realize that all this hard work is coming from you—nobody else but you. So when you hit your goal weight, you can say to yourself "I did this," "look at what I did," or "I can't believe how far I've come to this point" when you succeed. You shouldn't lose more than one to two pounds a week, otherwise you're just asking for trouble and most likely will put the weight back on.

You can do it. Just put in the effort, love your life, and appreciate yourself no matter what stage you're in, and always stay positive.

Remember to consult with you primary healthcare provider before starting any health or weight loss regimen.

References

http://www.marketwire.com/press-release/spending-on-weight-loss-products-to-reach-more-than-134-billion-in-2014-1354393.htm

Traditional Chinese Medicine (TCM) and Insomnia

In TCM, a common cause of of insomnia is due to disharmony of your heart qi/blood energy, which is also going to affect or be affected by the qi (chi) of another organ, such as the spleen qi/blood energy (responsible for digesting and metabolizing), kidney yin energy (responsible for growth and longevity), or the liver blood energy (responsible for promoting harmonious flow of qi throughout the body, also deals with emotions). By looking at your tongue, and feeling your pulse, we are able to get a better idea of what systems may be out of order in your body.

I suggest diving into resources that go more into detail about basic Chinese Medicine theory on organs and meridians and how we view the human body. What you will learn will be invaluable to your health.

Other suggestions that may help with insomnia:

- Physical activity and exercise throughout the day—no excuses.

- Meditation in the morning and an hour before you get to bed, 15 minutes each session.

- Counting backwards from 100 while breathing in slow and with soft breath.

- Avoid eating spicy foods in the evening.

- Bad digestion and GI problems can contribute to insomnia, so eating the right foods for your body type is important.

- Try drinking a small cup of chamomile tea in the evening.

Sleep and Susceptibility to Diabetes and Obesity

Diabetes, Sleep, and Your Health

– According to an article in the April 2012 issue of *Science* magazine, a study published in the *Journal of Science Translational Medicine* found that people may be priming themselves for diabetes and obesity due to a lack of sleep and irregular sleeping patterns. Those especially affected were young men, who had lowered their insulin response from only a week of reduced amounts of sleep[1].

Diabetes is a condition where the body is unable to metabolize sugar properly, which leads to excess glucose levels in the blood.

The study included 21 participants who received 5.6 hours of sleep a night, and went to sleep at different times to mimic a working individual with rotating shifts. The study found that people were more agitated when sleep deprived. Furthermore, the amount of glucose in the bloodstream was much higher in each person and three of the participants reached levels that the researchers called pre-diabetic.[2] Another interesting finding from researchers was the effects of sleeping depravity on the metabolic resting rate. Your metabolic resting rate represents the calories being burned on a normal everyday basis as you go about your day. The sleep deprived individuals were shown to have as much as an 8% reduction in their metabolic resting rates after a few weeks in the study. For those trying to lose weight or become leaner, that can be a big drag in your weight management efforts.

Sleep is IMPORTANT!

The article comments that this study demonstrates the important connection between disruption of the body's natural rhythm and the relationship to diabetes and obesity. In another study I found on pubmed.gov looking at over 3,000 individuals, shorter and longer durations of sleep cycles were associated with newly diagnosed diabetes, but not in pre-diabetics.[3]

I've always been an advocate of good sleep. Sound sleep will help you think better, keep you in a happy emotional state, and give you the energy you need to make it through a hard day. Since the downturn of the economy, many working individuals have picked up additional shifts to cover their costs, and many times at the cost of sleep. I understand completely, but just remember this equation: Good Sleep = Full Alertness = Ability to create new ways to solve problems.

If you're having trouble sleeping, acupuncture can be an effective treatment for insomnia and other sleeping disorders. You can find more information in my post on Acupuncture for Insomnia.

References

1,2. Leslie, M. 2012. Sleep study suggests Triggers for Diabetes and Obesity. *Science*. April 2012, pg143

3. Chi-Yuan Chao, Jin-Shang Wu, Yi-Ching Yang, Chi-Chen Shih, Ru-Hsueh Wang, Feng-Hwa Lu, Chih-Jen Chang. 2011.Sleep duration is a potential risk factor for newly diagnosed type 2 diabetes mellitus. *Metabolism – Clinical and Experimental* Volume 60, Issue 6 , Pages 799-804, June 2011

4. Sleep apnea predicts distinct alterations in glucose homeostasis and biomarkers in obese adults with normal and impaired glucose metabolism. *Cardiovasc Diabetol*. 2010; 9: 83.Published online 2010 December 1

The Importance of Breathing Exercises

Breathing is Life

Breathing is such a natural process that we do it without taking notice throughout the day. Everyone knows without breath there is no life, so breathing is the most vital mechanism needed for survival. The other would be, as you probably guessed, consumption of food and water. In Traditional Chinese Medicine, the basis for acquiring qi ("chee") into your body that keeps you alive involves obtaining qi from the air and qi from the foods consumed, and combining those two elements to create a form of energy that can be used and distributed to regulate all the body's natural biological functions.

So why is it important for us to improve our breathing habits?

Breathing gives us a way to communicate with the unconscious mind. Heart rate, digestive functions, circulation, and many other involuntary bodily functions can positively be affected by breathing. When we are stressed out, we are activating our sympathetic nervous system which affects how we react to situations and leaves us more in "guard" mode. Breathing helps to kick in the parasympathetic system, which helps us to relax and enjoy life.

Breathing exercises and deep breathing brings oxygen to the base of our lungs. There is a large amount of blood flow that occurs in the lower regions of the lungs, and shallow inhalation into the upper chest area causes your body to miss out on superb health benefits. Less oxygen is transferred into the blood system with shallow chest breathing and results in poor delivery of nutrients to tissues of the body.[1]

Yoga has been around for thousands of years, which means the exercise has undergone thousands of years of refinement. Pranayama, which is known as regulated breathing or the control of life/energy, has been shown to contain numerous benefits when practiced regularly. Benefits include decreased stress, cardiovascular improvement, improved respiratory functions, and pranayama helps to regulate and balance the autonomic nervous system.[2]

The Scientific Research on Breathing Exercises

In a study looking at fifteen (15) Hemodialysis patients, inspiratory muscle training was found to increase the walking distance of the individuals.[3]

Chronic Obstructive Pulmonary Disease (COPD) is a disease in which the airways of the lungs become obstructed, making it more difficult to breath. Chronic bronchitis and emphysema are two conditions that fall under this category. In a randomized control study examining COPD patients and breathing exercises, researchers found that respiratory exercises were effective in reducing fatigue in COPD patients.[4]

The Senobi breathing exercise is a combination of stretching and breathing techniques aimed at inducing calmness and relaxation, as well as promoting health and vitality. In a study examining 20 overweight women suffering from depression, the Senobi breathing technique was found to help with improving the depression as well as increasing the secretion of neurotransmitters and hormones such as Noradrenaline (Norepinephrine), Dopamine, 5-HIAA (breakdown byproduct of serotonin), Estradiol, and Growth Hormone.[5] So utilizing this breathing technique takes care of multiple systems in the body and can be safely integrated into your normal routine.

Breathing For Your Profession

Policemen, firefighters, health professionals, or anyone working long hours and having the responsibility of making tough decisions at any given moment can benefit from breathing techniques. Maybe you are on a team that is stuck in a mental rut and needs some type of motivation and clarity to progress forward. No matter what your needs may be, breathing techniques can help you be on top of your "A" game.

Breathing and Martial Arts

As a martial artist, deep breathing can be the key to remaining focused in any situation. In order to generate maximum power, the muscles should be kept loose and relaxed, ready to exert power at any given moment. How do we accomplish this? By breathing, and using different methods to strengthen our breathing techniques, such as meditation, having the correct breathing tempo when working out, and utilizing exercises, such as Qigong, that have been developed to maximize your breath and vitality.

Every Breath You Take Counts!

Listen, I put a lot of emphasis into breathing because there are many more benefits that I did not cover in this blog post that can be achieved through practice. If you are interested in learning proper breathing techniques, it is recommended that you learn from a trained professional who can get you started and make sure that you are doing the exercises correctly. Live, learn, enjoy life, and enjoy every breath taken!

Sources and References

1. Rakel, D. Faass, N. 2006. *Complementary Medicine in Clinical Practice*. Jones and Barlett Publishers, Inc.

2. Veerabhadrappa SG, Baljoshi VS, Khanapure S, Herur A, Patil S, Ankad RB, Chinagudi S. Effect of yogic bellows on cardiovascular autonomic reactivity. *J Cardiovasc Dis Res*. 2011 Oct-Dec; 2(4): 223–227.

3. Gomieiro LT, et al. Effects of inspiratory muscle training in hemodialysis patients. *J. Bras. Nefrol.* vol.33 no.1 São Paulo Jan./Mar. 2011

4. Zakerimoghadam M, Tavasoli K, Nejad AK, Khoshkesht S. The effect of breathing exercises on the fatigue levels of patients with chronic obstructive pulmonary disease. *Acta Med Indones.* 2011 Jan;43(1):29-33.

5. Sato K, Kawamura T, Yamagiwa S. The "Senobi" breathing exercise ameliorates depression in obese women through up-regulation of sympathetic nerve activity and hormone secretion. *Biomedical Research.* Vol. 32 (2011) No. 2 April P 175-180

Cinnamon for Your Health

The Healthy World of Cinnamon

Cinnamon is one of my favorite herbs and has many uses in Chinese herbology. It has been used for thousands of years for in the prevention and recovery from disease. The first thing that may come to mind for most people when they hear cinnamon is the word "roll," but what are some of the benefits associated with this powerful herb?

Cinnamon and Traditional Chinese Medicine Herbology

The Chinese name for the type of cinnamon twig used in Chinese Medicine is called Gui Zhi (pronounced GWAY Juh), and the pharmaceutical name is Cinnamomi Ramulus, according to the Materia Medica by Dan Bensky. In Traditional Chinese Medicine, cinnamon has the power to unblock what we call the yang qi and release the muscle layers. To give you a better understanding of what this means, your yang qi flows throughout your body and is responsible for warming and circulating throughout your body. Cinnamon has the power to open up your meridians, unblocking any energy roadblocks you may have. It is used in many herbal cold formulas, and some herbalists may use this for stroke recovery patients as well.

The Research on Cinnamon

There is research available on the benefits of cinnamon, including its potential role in managing diabetes and blood sugar levels, prevention of insulin resistance, and potential ability to induce tumor cell death in animal studies.[1] Particular amounts of cinnamon that were taken orally daily were shown to reduce serum glucose and lipid levels.[2] In one randomized controlled study, cinnamon had lowered the HbA1C level by 0.83%, as compared to what was called "usual care" at 0.37%3.

Cinnamon has also been shown to exhibit anti-inflammatory properties.[4]

There was one randomized controlled study that I found that concluded cinnamon did not have an effect on glucose or lipid levels.[5] This was conducted for six weeks with 25 postmenopausal type 2 diabetes patients.

It Takes the Whole Group

So before you go rushing to the store and spending all your money on the newest health supplement, just know that in Traditional Chinese Medicine herbs are very, very rarely prescribed alone. All herbs need to be combined in formulas and mixtures in order to regulate one another and work in harmony. In a clinical aspect, when cinnamon is prescribed by an acupuncturist, it will be combined in a formula that is for that particular patient, no one else. If you are interested in knowing if cinnamon would be beneficial to your health and holistic healing regimen, then you should go visit a local, licensed acupuncturist for guidance.

References:

1. Kwon HK, Hwang JS, So JS, Lee CG, Sahoo A, Ryu JH, Jeon WK, Ko BS, Im CR, Lee SH, Park ZY, Im SH.Cinnamon extract induces tumor cell death through inhibition of NFκB and AP1. *BMC Cancer.* 2010 Jul 24;10:392.

2, 3. W. Xie, Y. Zhao, Y. Zhang. Traditional Chinese Medicines in Treatment of Patients with Type 2 Diabetes Mellitus. *Evid Based Complement Alternat Med.* 2011; 2011:Published online 2011 March 17

4. Kwon HK, Hwang JS, Lee CG, So JS, Sahoo A, Im CR, Jeon WK, Ko BS, Lee SH, Park ZY, Im SH. Cinnamon extract suppresses experimental colitis through modulation of antigen-presenting cells. *World J Gastroenterol.* 2011 Feb 28;17(8):976-86

5. K. Vanschoonbeek, B.Thomassen, J. Senden, W. Wodzig. L. van Loon. Cinnamon Supplementation Does Not Improve Glycemic Control in Postmenopausal Type 2 Diabetes Patients. 2006. *American Society for Nutrition*

Qin B, Panickar KS, Anderson RA. Cinnamon: potential role in the prevention of insulin resistance, metabolic syndrome, and type 2 diabetes. *J Diabetes Sci Technol.* 2010 May 1;4(3):685-93.

D. Bensky, S. Clavey, E. Stoger. *Chinese Herbal Medicine Materia Medica.* 2004. Eastland Press, Seattle Wa

The Benefits of Stretching and Flexibility Training

Stretching and flexibility training is an area I've personally neglected over the past few weeks and I didn't realize what a hindrance it was creating in my training and health in general. I've always believed in the saying, "Increase range of motion, decrease pain," and always will, unless something else challenges my mind. Stretching can help decrease injury during martial arts training or sports play as well as increase your overall range of motion.

In the martial arts world, flexibility has always been an important aspect for training, as a flexible body can perform more complex maneuvers. Sometimes I think it is a neglected aspect due to the fact that martial arts are associated with flashy kicks and moves which may cause some people to focus more solely on the combative aspect, acquiring only the minimal amount of flexibility needed to execute a technique, such as the roundhouse.

There are many more benefits that come with increased flexibility and just to name a few, here are some.

1. Reduces Stress

This is a biggie. Here in the US, stress is a huge problem and it can literally ruin your life. So what is one way we can help to reduce the anger and anxiety that we're feeling? Stretch out the muscles and relax. Slow, deep breathing will bring more oxygen to the muscles and brain and balance the autonomic nervous system. Focused stretching will help elongate the muscles and stretch out the microfilaments (muscle fibers) and help with a longer, smoother muscle contraction.

2. Helps Your Muscles Become Stronger

The more muscle fibers you can recruit in a movement, the better. Making use of more fibers gives you better control over movement and more strength. In Kung Fu, for instance, there are many low stances performed during training and flexibility is the key to achieving the strength and stability to hold your stance. All martial arts styles require strong legs, and implementing a good flexibility training strategy can help in the long run.

It can make a big difference in how your legs feel when you walk and perform other exercises.

3. Gives You Better Posture and Control

Imagine being able to have more control over the ground you walk on. Imagine being able to improve the way you sit, stand, and look. Good posture plays an important role in maintaining good neuro-musculoskeletal health, projecting a sense of confidence and helping to combat the effects of aging.

To add a stretching and flexibility regimen into your workout, it's best to find knowledgeable guidance so that you don't hurt yourself or stretch improperly. Yoga, martial arts, ballet, and gymnastics are just some of the different activities that build up flexibility over time. The key is to find what works for you and get more than just those five seconds of holding your foot.

5 Ways to Help Prevent Spleen Qi Deficiency

Been overworking yourself lately? Haven't been eating right? Sleeping late? Well, congratulations, that's a great recipe for inducing what is known in Traditional Chinese Medicine as Spleen Qi deficiency. What is thaaaat, you ask? Well, let's find out.

From a Chinese Medicine standpoint, the spleen energetically controls the digestion and intake of foods consumed. It can be likened to the basal metabolic rate through a bio-medical perspective. It is partnered with the stomach, and both play a role in digestive activities in the upper half of your body. It also plays a role in muscle strength, blood production, and water metabolism.

From a bio-medical physiological standpoint, the spleen actually plays a role in immunity and red blood cell destruction, and it acts as a blood reservoir.1

Spleen Qi deficiency is usually one of the first signs of an internal disorder in Traditional Chinese Medicines. Symptoms can vary, but based on my experience, as well as from the book *Chinese Acupuncture and Moxibustion*, symptoms may include tiredness and fatigue, indigestion, a reduced appetite, and constipation.

Seeing this in the clinic often, I must say there are some tips that I've passed along to my patients which can have a positive impact in our overall health in the short term and long run.

1. Stop Stressing

You may hear this a lot, but it is the truth. When you have much on your mind, then it affects every aspect of your life. Constant worrying will affect your digestion and eventually affect your overall health. Also, yin and yang theory dictates that when one side is affected, the other side will be affected as well. So other organs such as the lung qi or the liver qi will be affected, which can end up having a snowballing effect on the body for years to come. Keep things positive no matter what and remember if you're ever down, there is only one other direction, which is up.

2. Do 30 Minutes of Walking a Day, Five Days a Week

Walking is a great exercise because it's easy to do, it's enjoyable, and it can help your body get into a relaxed state. Don't over strain yourself if you can't do it all at once. In fact, I enjoy breaking my walks up into 20 minutes in the morning and another 20 later on in the day. Exercise can make a world of a difference in your health condition. I've seen people with great nutrition habits skip out on the exercise, and that's a big missing component in achieving optimal health.

3. Eat Foods That Are Easily Digestible

In Chinese Medicine theory, we promote warmth in many ways, and eating warm meals is one of those. Soups are great for boosting the spleen qi since they're light and can be digested quickly. Steamed vegetables are great, and having a warm breakfast can boost your energy for the day.

Greasy and sweet foods are not your friends. Great to hang out with once in a while, but they're the type of friends that'll get you in trouble.

Is it wrong to have something cold when it's blazing hot? No. But sometimes here in society we just go waaay overboard and just go with the flow. Ice cold drinks year round? Especially in winter? If you want to slow down your qi extremely, then stuff your digestive system with the coldest foods you can find (don't do that, I was being sarcastic). It's not a good slow down either.

4. Eat in Peace

When was the last time you enjoyed a quiet meal without any distractions? As acupuncturists in school, we learned that eating while distracted can have a negative effect on the digestive qualities of your spleen qi. Watching TV, working on the computer, and eating while driving. We all have been victims to these habits, and is anyone perfect? No. But being aware of it and giving ourselves time to enjoy our meals will pay off big in the long run.

5. *Do Some Qigong*

I had to bring it up! What is Qigong? It is comprised of breathing exercises developed in China that are thousands of years old. Qigong masters are known to have excellent health and vitality. Tai Chi is a slow moving, meditative form of Qigong, hence many of the benefits are overlapping. However, Qigong gives you a chance to focus on and really synchronize your qi and breathing. Can you build your qi up? Yes. Can you move your qi? Yes, and actually you have all types of qi moving all the time. So Tai Chi Chuan and Qigong go hand in hand, and practicing both is recommended to achieve the maximum health benefits.

Good habits are huge benefits in life. Usually a person who is active will remain active, as in Newton's first law of motion: An object in motion will stay in motion.

How do you know if you have spleen qi deficiency? Only your acupuncturist could tell you that..and your diet.

Please do not self diagnose yourself and go see a licensed acupuncturist for health related concerns.

References:
1. Thibodeau, G. Patton, K. *Anatomy and physiology*. 2003
Chinese Acupuncture and Moxibustion, Cheng Xinnong, 1999
Photo Credit Top: © Julien Tromeur

Feeling the Stress Building Up? Beating the Anxiety Rush

Whether it's waiting to get through the last five minutes of class, or surviving a conversation with someone who strikes your fancy, finding ways to deal with anxiety can be a vital life skill.

Shaking your leg, or "shaky leg" as I like to call it, is a common habit when you're feeling anxious at the moment. You know what I'm talking about, the rapid up and down movement of the leg that comes from extreme annoyance or anxiousness to move. The back heel moving up and down as you're constantly looking at the clock or your watch.

In my acupuncture grad curriculum, we had classes that were sometimes four hours long, so devising strategies to defeat fatigue and anxiety became an acquired skill. Through personal experience and trial-n-error, I was able discover some very valuable techniques to help reduce stress at any given moment.

What are some of the ways I've found that may help calm down your anxious shaky leg or anxiousness in general? Sit tight, my friend. I bet you're anxious to find out the answer.

Breathing is Your Best Friend

Take three slow breaths in and out, utilizing abdominal breathing. Is the day moving so fast that you can't take 30 seconds to refresh your thought pattern and bring yourself into a more focused state? No, it's not, and it's totally worth it. If you find difficulty in finding time to taking a few breaths, then you know where to start.

Take More Walks Around the Building

Pent up energy can be expressed in many different ways, and taking a walking break around the building can help you to reduce that stress. Heck, do a five to 10 minute walk every hour to keep your blood pumping and at the same time reduce stress. Have time to squeeze in some push-ups? Bust out 20, do two minutes of deep breathing, and see if that helps you to relax and enjoy the situation.

If you catch yourself sighing often, we typically contribute it to stagnation of liver qi, which maintains the smooth flow of qi throughout your body and plays a role in keeping you emotionally stable. Sighing is a signal of blocked qi in the upper portion of your body that needs to be released, and is usually related with some type of personal concerns. This in turn can create anxiety in us during stressful situations. One of the ways to help move your qi and release tension is to take enjoyable walks.

Get Ready for the Stressful Event

Lastly, preparation is your best friend. We practice meditation so that we train the mind and body to be relaxed and work in synchronicity throughout the day. We work out our muscles so that they may become stronger and handle more weight. The same goes for training your patience. There are exercises you can do to strengthen your ability to stay focused and reduce fatigue when in a classroom, meeting, or any situation which requires paying attention.

This is just a small list of activities that you can do to help manage your anxiety in a stressful situation. Do you have any times where using any of these techniques could have helped you during a stressful event?

Remember to consult a healthcare professional if you feel that you are suffering from anxiety disorders, or neurological or psychological concerns.

Self Care Acupressure For Constipation and Better Digestion

If you've been experiencing bit of digestive difficulty or constipation, then maybe acupressure may help with getting things moving. I have personally used these points to help with, you know, doing the number "two," and I have experienced great results. You don't necessarily have to do this while on the commode, just massage these points to stimulate the digestive system any time you need a boost.

The Stomach Meridian

These points run along a meridian known as the stomach meridian. Just like in western physiology, the stomach meridian and organ deal with food storage and plays a role in digestion. Stimulation of these points can also help with indigestion, low energy, reduced appetite, and nausea.

This meridian runs one finger away, about one half to three quarters of an inch from the outside of your shin bone, as you can see from the picture below.

The stomach meridian begins on the face and ends at the toes. Many points exist that exhibit many types of positive effects not only for your digestive system but for your body as a whole. This simple acupressure technique focuses on only a small but powerful section of the meridian.

How to Do It

To stimulate the area, slightly rub down the muscle to the outside of your shin bone. Start about three inches below your knee and go down about halfway, then repeat. Massage the meridian downwards with your thumb and do this five times with each leg. Repeat the process again if you wish.

The acupuncture points that you're stimulating include points called Stomach 36, 37, and 39. Stomach-36 is a widely used point for building energy. Stomach-37 and Stomach-39 are associated with the large intestines and the small intestines in Chinese Medicine theory and can have a strong effect on these organs.

As you can imagine, almost the entire digestive system is affected. It is interesting how everything is inter-connected and multiple systems in the body need to be treated to obtain optimal wellness.

Here are a couple of points to keep in mind:

- You need to eat foods that can be easily digested and contain nutritional value. I'm a big fan of crock pots and soups. If you don't have one, you can easily get one for twenty bucks. Fill it up with all types of veggies, add some spices, and you're good to go.

- Don't overdo it. Smooth and relaxed is the key. We are helping to loosen up the muscle and it should feel less tense as you massage it.

- Clear your mind, don't think. Don't sit in anticipation waiting for something to happen, just breathe normally and calmly. For qi to flow freely and to experience the full benefits of acupressure, you must be relaxed and calm.

- This technique works well if you feel unfinished in the process of passing stools.

This is a natural way to help out your body if needed.

If you have any questions on how acupressure can help with other health conditions and diseases, contact an acupuncturist in your area.

What has been your experience with acupressure?

3 Ways to Help Eliminate Stress Now

Let's face it, being stressed out may be a buzzword, and yes, you know you're stressed, but come on, let's get real? You have real threats, like being low on funds or family problems that seem to have no solution. I understand, been there, still there. However, there are some things you can do to help de-stress yourself and bring about a more positive attitude. Why have a positive attitude? Because it can help you think outside the box, and from my personal experience there is nothing you can't get through when you feel positive and play the game of life to the best of your ability. So what can you do to help reduce the stress in your world?

1. Breathe!

Yes, breathe. Breathe slowly in through the nose and out through the nose, focusing your energy about an inch and a half below your belly button. This area is known as the Dan tian in Chinese Medicine and is considered an area important to life and vigor. If you can't take the time to stop and take three slow, relaxed, deep, controlled breaths, then that's the first problem. Don't let life go so fast that you can't slow yourself down and give yourself time to center your qi ("chee"), your focus, or bring your body to a level of homeostasis.

2. Take a 10 Minute Walk

Laps around the block or your building can give you more energy and improve your mood. Don't waste your ten minute break at work, do something productive like getting rid of the built up tension. Maybe you have tension with your boss or co-workers (or maybe you are the boss with lousy employees!) or you had an argument with your spouse, and taking some time to walk is what you need. 10 minutes is only the minimum; you can go for 15 or

20 if you feel like it. Walking can help move your qi and get your energy moving, especially when you hit that afternoon energy drop when you want to go to sleep. Keep it moving!

3. Use Preventative Medicine

Did you know that you don't have to wait until you are broken down to see an acupuncturist? Holistic therapies such as acupuncture focus on preventing disease and helping the body to become as strong as possible. In Traditional Chinese Medicine, mild stress can be considered the early point of disorder in the body, and it can either get better or get worse. If financial burden is an issue, try to find a community acupuncture clinic in your town or find an acupuncturist that offers sliding rates or discounted health services.

What Is Stress?

According to physiologists, stress is any stimulus that directly or indirectly stimulates neurons of the hypothalamus to release corticotropin-releasing hormone (CRH), which then initiates many diverse changes in the body.[1] In plain English, that means anything that causes us to react in a certain way. This is known as the stress response.

Hans Selye of McGill University was one of the pioneer researchers of stress. His research led him to believe that the body exhibits certain responses when confronted with an outside stimulus or threat. In today's society, we are constantly bombarded with stressors that keep us on edge. This is why we must learn to identify our stressful interactions and deal with them accordingly.

There are many other ways to help you reduce the stress and anxiety in your life, so please don't feel limited just to the ideas I have suggested here. The more you begin to think and find a solution, the better off you will be in the long run.

1. Thibodeau, G. *Anatomy and Physiology*, Mosby Inc, 2003

About the Author

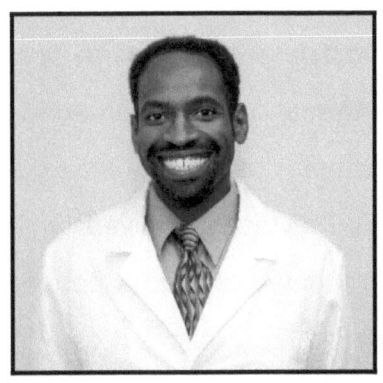

Hi, my name is Carlo and I graduated with a Masters in Acupuncture and Oriental Medicine from Southern California University of Health Sciences in 2009 and became licensed in California in 2011. Prior to completing my studies in Chinese Medicine, I completed my Bachelor's of Science in Business Management from Cal Poly Pomona and afterwards decided to pursue deeper into the health sciences.

I have over fourteen years of experience in health and general wellness. In addition, I have been studying the martial arts for over 10 years, primarily in the styles of Eagle Claw Kung Fu, Long Fist Wushu, Yang and Hao style Tai Chi Chuan, Qigong, No-gi Jujitsu and submission grappling.

My journey into health began when I lost over 55 pounds my sophomore year in college. It was a big accomplishment in my life and from then on I decided to always find new ways to keep healthy. However, I wanted to take it a step further and stay healthy through natural exercises and nutrients.

It is not easy sometimes to rid ourselves of ailments that may drag us down, but step by step and day by day you can move towards the healing process.

Acknowledgements

I hope you enjoyed this book and please know that many more are on the way. I share what I know, and I have learned from some of the best. Thank you first to my parents for their guidance and wisdom. Thanks to California Polytechnic University, Pomona for providing me with an excellent undergraduate experience. To Southern California University of Health Sciences (Los Angeles College of Chiropractic), Whittier for providing me with the education, knowledge, and skill set to become a competent and caring practitioner. Finally, thanks to all of my martial arts instructors, for your knowledge has helped me to achieve what I have.

To learn more about my bio or about my clinic, please feel free to visit my website www.csjacupuncture.com.